LET'S NOT GET FAT

HOW TO CHANGE YOUR PERSPECTIVE ABOUT LIVING A FIT AND HEALTHIER LIFESTYLE IN ORDER TO TRULY REACH YOUR BREAKTHROUGH

NATE ANDRES

CONTENTS

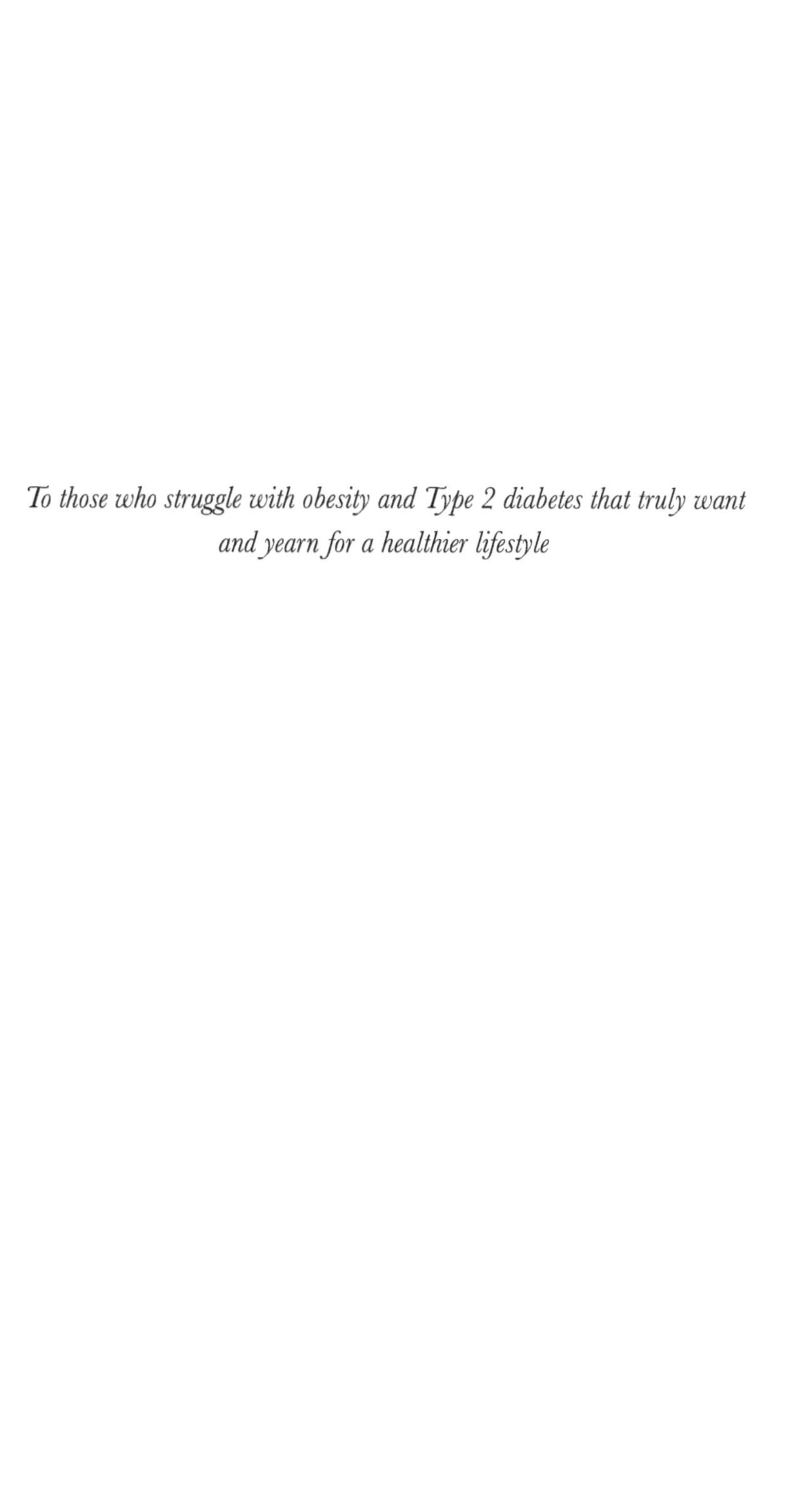

To those who struggle with obesity and Type 2 diabetes that truly want and yearn for a healthier lifestyle

ACKNOWLEDGMENTS

Mom, Dad, Melina & Bianca

CHAPTER 1

THE WORLD DOESN'T CARE ABOUT YOUR FEELINGS

Disclaimer: If you are a person that does not like being opened minded about different ways of thinking and different perspectives to better oneself, then this book should probably be gifted to one of your friends that is.

Anyways, I know you are probably thinking, "Oh my God, why does this book's title already tick me off?" Or "Why the fuck am I even reading this in the first place?"

I just want to say- I totally feel for you. It is not my intention whatsoever to put any human being down about their weight or maybe their insecurities. Because they are real. However, what my intentions actually are is to help whoever reads this book to finally provide them the tools to breakthrough their current lifestyle in order to live in their more ideal lifestyle that they always envision themselves in. So if that is you, I am ecstatic to say that you are reading this at the right place at the right time and I couldn't be more excited for you.

With that said, let's get this party started.

So who am I anyways? Who is this person that is trying to supposedly guide me down a path to a healthier and much more fit lifestyle? Well, for starters, my name is Nate. I have been working out at a relatively intense level for about 8 years in a row. I have competed in several workout and combat competitions, most of them being CrossFit competitions. I have won third in the world for the 2013 Reebok CrossFit Kids Games when I was 14 years old being the smallest one in my age class. I am filipino so I was never a very built person with mass and natural strength.

Now 8 years later, I serve as a coach at CrossFit Live helping others reach their desired health and fitness lifestyle. I have also ventured into various different types of exercise including gymnastics, calisthenics, parkour, and straight olympic weightlifting. I have also started my own modern advertising business to help other individuals and businesses reach their goals and ideal lifestyles outside of the gym as well.

I remember always being the scrawny asian kid, never able to lift up a penny and always getting picked on at school and sports. I never found any type of motivation to become more well-rounded and fit because I sort of accepted that how I am is how I am. But once I realized that those were just excuses and it's only up to me to see if I have a shot of becoming a better version of myself, I began my journey, just as you will right now.

As much as I want to let you know that this journey towards your health and fitness is going to be a piece of cake, I can't. Not even close. It will be one of the hardest tasks you will perform in your lifetime because this is a journey, not a process. The difference? A process ends. A journey doesn't. I always reference reaching your ideal lifestyle and not your ideal goal is because after you reach a goal, it's accomplished. But when you reach a lifestyle, it's maintenance. Yes, 90% of the game will be to maintain your lifestyle. But it's okay, you'll learn to love it soon.

So what are you going to get out of this book that you won't find in any other fitness book? Easy. Alongside all the practical value like dieting, exercising tips, etc, we're going to add something that not a lot of books do. We're going to suffocate all of our bullshit. "Wait, I don't have any bullshit." Bullshit. Everyone does. The first step to solve a problem is to realize that there is one. And if we can't accept that we have bullshit, guess where the bullshit is going to sit until you do… inside yourself as fat and lack of general stamina. And I and your loved ones don't want that for you.

Funny that I mention bullshit- notice how my grammar, language, ideas aren't so "formal" or "politically correct"? Welcome to step 1. This is not only because I suck at writing, but most importantly, to get you to to see through the surface level. If you actually can't see the true intentions in someone just because they didn't grammatically format paragraphs how they teach in college, then go and read one that does. But I hope that you can see through that and see the true value in this book and the true intentions to actually get your life in a truly better position regardless of the surface level shortcomings.

Take this book cover for example. It could be seen as an insult to many. I understand that. But I want to see who is willing to look past that with hopes to find something that may better themselves. Because I can guarantee that if I named the book: Let's Get Healthy- all that will go through your mind is, "Yeah, yeah, yeah." The true problem hasn't been addressed. And i a problem isn't addressed, it can't be solved.

This goes into something that most fitness people don't talk about. Self-awareness. What do I mean? Not everyone wants to be Dwayne "The Rock" Johnson or Michael B. Jordan. As much as society would love to assume so, I have empathy that everyone has different goals for themselves-different ideal lifestyles, and it makes sense. Everyone has different ages, ambitions, desires, etc. Someone who is 18 reading this may want to look like Zac Efron but a 47 year old lady probably won't.

Self-awareness is key. Know exactly what you want from yourself. I'm 19 years old currently and I know I want to push myself to the maximum everyday. Only because that's where my ambition takes me. But for those of you who just want to stay mobile and lose weight enough to play with your grand-kids, I respect that. So throughout this book, feel free to adjust anything to cater to your ideal lifestyle- but don't get that twisted with excuses. There is a very fine line so I'm counting on you to hold yourself accountable to really push yourself to reach your true and genuine goal.

This book isn't meant to be long either. This book is meant to be as long as it needs to be in order to provide you with as much necessary value as possible. I say necessary because a lot of books and courses tend to put, what I like to call "fluff", into their products to give the illusion that the more and longer it is, the more value. That's just not true. I want to be straight up and give you all the necessary tools and knowledge to close this book as soon as you can in order to reach your breakthrough once and for all because i know life is short and you don't have all the time in the world to read "fluff". So let's do this shall we?

The World Really Doesn't Care

When we complain that life is hard, the cars on the freeway still drive. When life hits us hard, the windmills in the fields still turn. I'm not saying you don't have real shit to deal with, we all do. But what I am saying is that the moment we become a victim of our shit, we let it have control over us.

If this still isn't coming clear, don't beat yourself up for it. This signifies the first aspect of achieving your ideal health and fitness lifestyle. Mindset. I know the word "mindset" gets thrown around a lot, tends to be very cliche. I get it. But the reality is that mindset ultimately plays 80% of the entire game. The other 20% being physical action. But why?

Take for example the first phrase: The World Doesn't Care About Your Feelings. It's a hard pill to swallow. But if you don't swallow it, the pill will continue to be there holding you down until you do. On top of that, the world ultimately doesn't care if you swallow it or not. To sum it up, the only way to actually push through the difficult times, to power through your breakthrough is to have yourself alone swallow these so called "pills" that keep you from getting to your goal.

By your keeping yourself accountable and progressively stop making excuses for yourself, the smoother the path will be to getting where you want to go.

The reason why there aren't a lot of people who make this breakthrough for themselves is because of this alone. After someone watches a motivational workout video and says to themselves, "Alright, let's lose this weight." but then feels pity for themselves after they do 5 sit-ups and gets tempted with freezing their fat off instead, it becomes a very hard task for someone to hold themselves to.

But the moment you realize within yourself that, "Hey you know what, no one is going to lose this fat for me and the world honestly doesn't care if I do it for myself, I have to do this and actually pull through.", the results will be insane.

Now this is where most people that hear this tip fail. They get introduced the self-accountability aspect but then two days later working on their new lifestyle, they end up like, "Man, this is hard." Now this is where I would normally say "No shit." But let me reiterate what this book is supposed to help you do: How to change your perspective.

Perspective is everything. Period. Everything in life is perspective. This is what I really want to pound you with because it is such a pivotal aspect in this whole mindset aspect.

Perspective, in short, is realizing that when your shirt gets dirty, you either say, "Damn it, my shirt is dirty now." Or, you stop yourself and say, "Well, at least this thing kept me warm today." Same shirt different perspective. Same concept with your health and fitness. If you look at difficulties as things to avoid, you will forever be miserable. However, once you learn to shift your perspective and seek difficulties and adversity, then you are going to see your ideal lifestyle real soon I can tell you that.

But Nate, why would I want to seek difficulties if they're hard?

Learn To Love Losing

I'm super glad I hypothetically asked that. Why? Because this is one of the most important perspectives to have especially in regards to your journey to becoming more fit and healthy. Really. I'm being straight up. Here's why: losing = growth. Therefore, if you like losing, you get growth. But if you don't like losing, there won't be as much growth. It's pretty simple, but I can see why it goes over 90% of people's head. Because they agree. But when they are actually in the moment of adversity, they forget it and complain. That alone will keep you from getting yourself where you want to go.

If hating pain slows you down, like it.

However, it is easier said than done. Afterall, avoiding pain is a part of human nature. Like, how does one actually learn to love pain and losing? One word, practice.

To get a little bit more practical… next time you feel the urge to drink that can of coke, or whatever your weakness is, and you keep yourself from drinking it and it hurts, remember that feeling, and realize that if you were to like that feeling, that coke won't have anything against you anymore. Still cloudy in the head? Let's simplify it. You're doing squats and you hate the pain in your legs. Next time you feel that, say to yourself, "I like it." It will feel weird at first, but the more you do it, the more you actually will like it. This is called conditioning. Conditioning doesn't just pertain to physical exercise, it pertains to the mind too.

But let's say you don't do it. You feel the pain and you let it get the best of you. So now you avoid it. But by avoiding it that requires you to push yourself less. Push yourself less = progress? We all wish, right?

I feel you, it is very difficult. But it is a barrier that you have to face inside yourself if you truly want to breakthrough to a better lifestyle.

So this is the type of perspective that I want you to have.

Working out shouldn't be something that you dread, but it should be something dreadful, that you seek. I know learning to love losing isn't really something that you do on a daily basis especially in the society that we live in today. Losing, in today's, terms is obviously used in a negative connotation very commonly. This is where I really want to emphasize the aspect about changing your perspective about working out. not only just working out but also with just living a healthier lifestyle. because for most people living a healthier lifestyle isn't something that everyone in America looks forward to doing. most people try to fight for comfort and ease. But if you think like everyone, you're going to be like everyone. And that's just the reality.

This is going to be the turning point to where you are going to start to develop a different mindset than the rest of society. if you manage to do that you will start to understand how important it is to start thinking differently and order to get different results. Yes, it does sound very cliche and very common sense. But common sense isn't so common anymore.we have to start to learn how to love to lose. since exercise and going on a diet will consist of a lot of pain and difficulty if we refuse to learn how to love to lose, we are subconsciously making our path rougher than it needs to be. I don't want to make this sound like some bullshit just to make you think a certain way and like me. This is very practical. If your mind has total control of over your body, doesn't it make sense to put the health and wellness of your mindset on the highest pedestal? It's all foundation.

Practice. Practice. Practice. Any chance you get to experience some sort of physical and mental adversity whether it's being more patient or doing 2 more pushups than usual, love it. Own it. Embrace it. I promise you that it will be one of the most life-changing adjustments you make in your life.

Motion = Emotion

Alright, let's get even more real here. This is an inevitable rollercoaster. There will be downtimes when sometimes, our mind isn't there our results are suffering for it. What do we do then?

This is the back up plan: Motion = Emotion. When you wake up and you just don't feel motivated to do anything and all you can think about are doughnuts, remember this. Motion = Emotion. Here's what I mean.

Have you ever been in a bad mood, grumpy, annoyed about everything? And then you see a cute video of a puppy on Instagram and you automatically change moods and say, "Fuck, that's cute." Yeah, those times. Those times are very similar to what I'm about to explain to you.

When you force your body to do certain things, your mind tends to follow. So if I were to ask you, "How would you describe someone who is depressed?" You would say, "Slouched, short of breath, small range of motion, etc." But if I were to ask you how would someone look if they were happy, it would be the total opposite. So what if you were to adjust your physical chemistry alone Take for example when you wake up in the morning and you're just groggy because you slept too much but you don't want to be, you drop down and do 10 pushups. Now, all of a sudden you are wide awake ready to do whatever is next when 15 sec ago you're mind was like "Fuck everything, I'm tired." This is what I'm trying to get at.

When your mind isn't there, use your body. Use your motion. If your mind really doesn't want to do the daily workout but you know you have to, without hesitation get something started and the rhythm will make your mind follow. Then the result you wanted has been done.

This is very difficult though. 95% of people will just let their mind take over because it's easier. But just realize that after this book, 99% of this whole journey will be all you. Not me, not your mom. Just you. It is completely up to you whether or not you will allow your mind to take over. But if you are someone who won't put up with that shit and are actually hungry for that breakthrough, make that body move, get into motion and keep moving forward.

One thing I do every morning, especially the groggy ones, is drop down and do 100 push-ups. Now, I'm not saying do this specifically, but do something. It's harder than it seems. Especially 3 months down the line and your mind starts to say, "Yeah yeah, motion = emotion." and then you fall asleep again for the fourth time. Really hold yourself accountable. Don't let your own mind be the reason you will never break-through to your ideal lifestyle.

CHAPTER 2

REWIRE YOUR BODY

Although the main purpose of this book is to change your perspective about ultimately living a healthier lifestyle, I want to really try to provide as much practical value that you can physically apply in your life so that when you close this book, you can actually have practical knowledge on what to do for your fitness life.

So now you know that this isn't going to be an easy path, you know what type of mindset it requires you to have- so now what? I'm going to be sharing you the practical knowledge that you can actually apply in your daily life to produce results. What are we going to start with first? Exercise.

This aspect of living a healthy life could be very broad. There are so many types of exercises, misconceptions about certain exercises, and virtually everything else that falls on that line. So let's take it one step at a time. Misconceptions.

There are a lot of misconceptions about exercises that

steer everyone in so many different directions. And I don't blame them. The options you can take on yourself are endless. Zumba, Pilates, ultrarunning, CrossFit, personal training, Orange Theory, etc. It's insane on how many different types of physical exercise regimens and routines there are available in the world. But I'm not here to talk about which one to pick. Instead, I'm going to tell you the science and requirements your body needs to go through in order to lose fat and get fit. That's why you're here right? Not to be told what type of exercise to do but to be informed on how to actually achieve the result you're striving for. So let's start off with the basics.

How Does Fat Leave the Body Anyways?

In order to figure out what we need to do to lose fat, we need to understand how fat leaves the body first. The only way fat leaves the body is by the result of a calorie deficit. I'm pretty sure you heard of the saying, "burning calories". Well, to go a little deeper, after you burn those calories and you continue to need more energy to perform your hard tasks, a.k.a. Exercises, your body uses the energy from its stored fat. The body then takes the stored fat, converts it into energy, then leaves the body.

But wait, how does the fat even leave the body if it's fat? Multiple ways. Sweat, urine, and the most interesting one, your breath. Yes, that carbon dioxide you exhale? That's fat leaving the body. Why am I telling you this? Because this is where it gets fun. If fat only naturally leaves the body through sweat, urine, and carbon dioxide, guess what we need to be doing a lot of? Drinking a lot of water and exercising in a high-intensity fashion that makes you sweat bullets and breathe like there's no tomorrow. Crazy, huh?

But the crazy thing is, is that those were all things we already knew what we needed to do before. We all know drinking lots of water was healthy for us but we still chose soda. We all knew that pushing ourselves in a high intensity fashion is good for our exercise but we choose to call it a day the moment we barely break a sweat. And we wonder why we aren't getting the results we want.

Now that we understand the foundation of how fat leaves our bodies, what do we physically do to actually make that happen?

Intensity Is the Measurement

Like I said in the beginning of the book, this is all predicated on how ambitious you are, what your true ideal goals are without using it as an excuse, etc. But I will speak on the behalf of the sole fact of losing fat and the best and most efficient way to do it. So here we go.

What is intensity anyways? I'm pretty sure we all know the basic idea around intensity but to provide a little more context, intensity is power. Power as in, force multiplied by distance, then divided by time. But for short, intensity is doing more work, faster.

Scary? It could be to most, but that's why most are still seeking results. It's scary. No worries though, it's said that the more you know about something, the less scarier it is. It gives you more certainty. So let's get certain.

What do I mean by intensity is the measurement? What I mean is that the amount of intensity you put into your exercise regimen equals the amount of fat you will lose over a certain period of time. For instance, if you jog a mile three times a week for 4 weeks, you will lose approximately the same amount of fat if you were to sprint 200 meters 5 times a day for only three times in one week. Now this is not an exact comparison, this is solely for demonstration purpose, but you get what I mean?

The amount of intensity equals the amount of fat you will lose over a period of time. So if that's the case, what do I do exactly? There are multiple things you can do.

Low Intensity Exercise

I wanted to include low intensity exercises for a couple reasons. One, not everyone's goal is to kill themselves physically everyday while some do. Two, it provides a type of progression to where maybe those who understand long-term know that they aren't capable of going too intense right now but eventually would want to.

So for low intensity exercises and workouts, these will be the basic workouts you would see on a daily basis. Zumba, Pilates, sitting exercises, all that good stuff. Anything that will give you a sweat, but not necessarily gasping for air on the floor like you're going to die.

This isn't to degrade any of these workouts however, this is to just state which workouts lie one the lesser intense side of the spectrum for those who are looking for something to fit their ambitions.

If you are completely new to physical activity and you really want to start working your way up from maybe an injury, health condition or etc, these are perfect starting points to keep on your list.

However, there is one thing about low intensity exercises that tend to consume most people and probably 90% of you who read this book will give into as well. That is comfortability.

Comfortability is your worst enemy when you are trying to live a healthier and fitter lifestyle. Why? Because living that lifestyle is supposed to be hard. And comfortability and difficulty are mutually exclusive meaning they can't both be present at the same time.

Another trait comfortability does to you is that it messes with your mind. Think of it this way, being comfortable is like preparing and tilling a garden for excuses. It starts to change the chemistry in your head to where you begin to believe that you are fine where you are and you don't need to push yourself as hard anymore. You will believe it. Even if you don't believe me now, trust me, it gets you.

So that would be my ultimate caution while entering the territory of low intensity exercises. Again, they're not bad exercises, if anything, they are good stepping stools. But they do come along with a lot of temptations to become comfortable and that's not what you want.

High Intensity Exercise

Greg Glassman, the CEO of CrossFit Inc. once said in 2002, " Be impressed by intensity, not volume." In other words, what Glassman was trying to say was to do more work in less time rather than more work in more time. Why though? Why does intensity hold such a high pedestal in this book? The reason being is because there are endless benefits scientifically and mentally. You burn more fat, you build a physically stronger heart, speeds up your metabolism and become more fit overall. A 2006 study from McMaster University states that after 8 weeks after doing high intensity workouts, subjects could bicycle for twice as long as they could have before the study.

So what do we have to have in order to do perform at this level? Honestly, a pair of lungs and a body. There is no super expensive equipment, machines, etc to perform at a high intensity level. All you need is yourself and the will to push yourself.

Some examples of high intensity workouts include Cross-Fit, Intensity, P90x, etc. But for most people, this could even start at home by yourself.

For example, next time you decide to go on your 2 mile run, try estimating how far 100 meters is from you and sprint to that point and back with all your might. Do that 3 times and I guarantee you will feel like you had a more effective workout than the full 2 miles from only 600 meters. Again, this is assuming that you want to lose fat. If you just want to have a jog because it's your way of getting a breath of fresh air, do it. But if you're trying to breakthrough a point in your life that you never reached before and want to actually lose the fat that's been taunting you all these years, start to prepare yourself with a lot of intensity.

Weightlifting

There are a lot of misconceptions about pumping the ol' iron at the gym. Bench presses, bicep curls, lateral pulls, shoulder presses, all the good stuff. Have you ever been in the position, or seen a friend that has, where you lift weights 24/7, hoping to get cut and ripped, but instead you only get bigger muscles and not necessarily the "cut" look you wanted? There's a reason why.

Think of it this way: In regards to fitness, your body is only made up of a ratio between muscle and fat. So when you strictly lift weights, you are only enhancing your muscle side. Meanwhile, your fat side is staying stagnant, in some cases getting worse. Why? There is no intense cardiovascular aspect. Sure, getting a new bench max may seem "intense" but your breathing is relatively normal still. You're not gasping for air.

Remember from early on in the book, fat leaves the body through breath, sweat, and urine. I guess you got the urine part down, but what the other two? Overtime, that adds up and all the fat around your now bigger muscles is still there.

So what's the solution? Stop lifting weights? Not at all. Lifting weights isn't the bad thing, but the imbalance is. Make sure that the more you lift weights, the more your need for cardio exercise grows as well.

CHAPTER 3

FUELING YOUR TANK

Growing up as a scrawny kid, I never felt the need to diet. I usually was that kid that had the fastest metabolism and ate whatever I wanted. But then as the years went by, I realized two things. The first, probably the most obvious, it doesn't always stay that way. We all heard of the freshman fifteen and the college years. That's just the way it is. But the second thing is for more of the youngins. The ones who don't feel like they need to eat healthy, which I don't blame them. I was the same way exactly. But if your ambition is high and you want to be above average, here's why it would matter.

Even though I knew within myself that even if I ate healthy, I would just get hungry again and there would be no difference. There is one difference however. That difference is the difference in energy.

Have you ever heard of a food coma? Or better yet, had

one? Yeah, remember that time and remember what you ate. That's what I mean.

When we eat unhealthy, it makes us feel groggy and slow. Once I realized this, I knew that I wouldn't be able to live up to my ambitions. I knew that I wouldn't be able to perform at my best and being the kid I was and still am, my competitive side came out. I knew that if I didn't adjust what I ate on a daily basis, everyone else that did would surpass me when I could've did something about it beforehand.

Not only will adjusting your diet give you more energy, it also takes you off the path of future or maybe even current health conditions.

In 2015, almost 10% of the entire American population had Type 2 diabetes. And by that prevalence rate, the amount of people with both type 1 and 2 diabetes will increase 54% by 2030.

I realized that even though I could have the excuse within myself that I have fast metabolism and I probably won't ever be apart of that statistic, very quickly I realized that I was not safe. The moment I would stop caring about what I eat, I could literally feel my body softening up and becoming physically weaker. I will never forget that moment and my job now is to make sure that you don't fall into the comfortability within that territory.

So what can we do?

I felt like the best and most efficient way to give as much value and context as possible around this subject is to start with the foundations, one food type at a time.

Carbs

There are a lot of misconceptions about carbs. "Carbs are bad for you.", "I'm cutting carbs out of my diet." and a lot more. Believe it or not, there are good carbohydrates out there that can actually provide a benefit to your health in the form of energy. These are called complex carbs. Some examples of complex carbohydrates include brown rice, sweet potatoes, quinoa, bananas, wheat bread and a lot more.

Typically you would eat a portion of cars alongside with a protein and some veggies. But these types of carbs will give you healthy, natural energy that your body could actually utilize. As you know, there are carbs out there that the body can't directly use and just treats it as fluff. These are called simple carbohydrates. Most commonly and unfortunately, what most of us do is consume these "fluff" carbs and not do any type of exercise. Where does it go? Gets thrown straight into the fat converting machine and gets stored. Do I even need to list these carbs? White rice, white bread, pasta, soda, pastries, breakfast cereal, all the good stuff.

So if you want to make a big difference into losing fat, start making those substitutions. It will be very hard, so maybe start off small. Eat a lot of brown rice? Substitute it with brown rice. Order wheat bread at your favorite sandwich place if they provide it. It won't be the best tasting decisions, but in the long run, it will be the best looking one.

Protein

Protein has a specific role in your journey to living a more fit lifestyle. What protein does for you is that when you exercise, more specifically with weights and new movement, it repairs the naturally torn muscle and acts as a recovery catalyst with the use of its amino acids. So basically, after you workout, protein helps your muscles recover.

What type of protein should we be consuming to get those recovery results? There are a lot of sources of protein you can consume but some may stand slightly healthier and more beneficial than others.

For example, meats. Meats such as steak, chicken breasts an even fish meat have tons of protein in them. Other sources of non-meat protein that still hold the same effect include beans, hemp seeds, quinoa, greek yogurt, and edamame.

But for most, people tend to choose meat. For meat however, there are some that could provide more of a health benefit than others. Typically you want meats that are lean with no fat. Yes, sorry, less flavor, but a better choice. This is like plain chicken breasts, steak, etc. Also, it doesn't help if the meat is fried of greased like fried fish or fresh greasy bacon. Although those tend to taste the best. Everything goes down to how bad you want that lifestyle.

So let's say you workout and for most of us, we don't

always have a thick slab of chicken breast for us to eat and recover our muscles. Are there any alternatives.

As you might see a lot of others take protein shakes right after their workout. That tends to be more convenient- I even have myself resort to that a lot of the times. However, just know that a chicken breast or a lean piece of steak will be the purest and most natural source of protein you can get as for protein shakes contain a lot of different chemicals, artificial flavorings, and all these other ingredients that we tend to not give a shit about but we know it's not natural.

Although these substitutions and different shifts of foods could taste less flavorful, seem more bland or maybe even make us give up, keep in mind what the whole purpose is. You have to recover, you have to stay on the grind if you want it bad enough. It is a puzzle piece to complete the entire puzzle which is your ideal lifestyle. And if you don't adjust it, you will know in the back of your head that you're not doing 100% of the things you could do to be where you want to be.

Veggies

As we all probably heard at one point in our lives, veggies are good for us. But how good are they really? Most of us refuse to include veggies into our daily intake of foods, but only because we don't really know much about their health benefits beyond that, "they're good for us."

When we choose our vegetables to include in our daily

meals, there are a couple things we should keep in mind to maximize the effectiveness of our portions and ultimately to keep in mind just for our motivation to maintain our inclusion of vegetables in our diet.

Did you know that the more green and leafy vegetables are the ones that hold the most health benefits for our bodies? Take spinach for example. Spinach is one of the super veggies that we can include in our meals. Some like it, some don't. But nonetheless, spinach is still unbelievably healthy. One cup (30g) of raw spinach provides 56% of your daily vitamin A, contains high amounts of beta-carotene and lutein, which are antioxidants that are associated to decreasing the risk of cancer and also contribute to lowering blood pressure and improving heart health.

Wow, just from a cup of fucking spinach. I get that you may or may not like spinach but lucky for you, there are an endless amount of veggies out there to choose from. You got carrots, broccoli, garlic, brussel sprouts, kale, peas, asparagus, and on and on and on. I'm not going to give a whole lecture on how each of them are beneficial for you, but I do have a little perspective I want to share.

Veggies aren't the most flavorful. But instead of complaining and tweeting about how disgusting they are, is there something we can do about it? Of course there fucking is. Make it taste better. Believe it or not, there are a lot of healthy spices, flavoring, and mix-ins to make your veggie intake more bearable.

What I tend to do is make some substitutions with some

of the typical seasonings and mix-ins like switching salt to sea salt making it less processed. Maybe switching cheese gratings on your broccoli with chopped garlic. These are small things I managed to do to make a huge difference to my vegetable intake and are definitely tangible things you can do too.

Keeping the Ball Rolling

Alright, we all know it's easy to read these delicious substitutions and get excited about them. But let's be real. How is all this effort and determination going to look like five months from now? The same? A little less? Giving in to those sodas here and there? Of course. It happens to everyone, including myself. So how do we stay on course.

One thing that I would highly recommend is meal prepping. I know, I know, meal prepping is for fitness freaks that have all the time in the world. That's actually not true. You don't hope for the time and energy, you make it. And for all the time you spend not believing that, there won't be any change, no matter how much you hope for it.

How would you start meal prepping? There are a couple ways. You can hire someone else or a business to do it for you or you can do it yourself. Most people do it themselves to save money.

What you typically want in your meal preps are a portion of protein, veggies and complex carbs in each meal. You can mix and match to make it more interesting as time goes on, trust me, you will want to. There are so many amazing recipes on the internet and YouTube to inspire you as well.

Another thing, that I do at least, is keep in mind the results. It's hard to stay determined to something that doesn't have it's purposed reinforced. Maybe like your job, or school, or hobbies. Same concept. Stay on the grind long enough to at least see the results. Once you see it, remember how that feels. Engrave in your head of the feeling you get when you look in the mirror and you see yourself getting that much closer to your goal.

It's an amazing feeling, use that as your fuel to keep the grind moving.

CHAPTER 4

LOOK TO YOUR LEFT AND RIGHT

We're going to start getting real practical now. This section is about a very underrated topic in the health and fitness world that is super pivotal and important as you go along your path.

Imagine you are running to your goal. That ideal lifestyle, that ideal body type you've always wanted, that diet that you plan to keep, maybe your workouts are getting more intense than ever but you seem to like it even more.

And as you're running there, you're running faster than ever and what I want you to imagine is who is running with you to your left and to your right? It may be people you know that are running to the same goal, the same direction as you, and maybe some strangers. Some of them may be role models that you haven't even met before. But who are they? Really try to think of that very thoroughly. Who is running with you in the same direction.

The purpose of this exercise is to become aware of which

people in your life are best supporting you towards your goal. Who is just as ambitious? Who has the same fitness desires as you? Once you figure out who they are, are they in your inner circle? Are they consistently in your life making a consistent impact for your greater good? These are the questions that we will be asking ourselves throughout the duration of this chapter and it's only going to get more and more real.

The Inner Circle

Some of you may have heard this phrase "inner circle". In this specific context it means the people you surround your-self with on a daily basis. It may be your immediate family, grandparents, guardians, friends, family-friends, classmates, coworkers, even people you follow on social platforms as well.

There's this saying that I'm pretty sure you might have heard of, "You are the sum of the five closest people in your life." Those five people especially, they are going to play a huge part in your journey whether you believe it or not.

Why am I putting so much emphasis on this concept? Because if those five to ten people eat like shit and you know you don't want to but there's so many of them that your dream and ideal lifestyle just gets overridden and you give in every single time. It happens everyday.

Even though this may seem like common sense, the most cliche tends to be the most difficult. Because obviously you care about them. Your friends aren't freaking pests or anything, but they might not have the same goals as you, which is totally fine. But what are you going to do about it?

Self-Awareness is Everything

I physically cannot read your mind, know 100% of the context of your life through the pages of this book. I just can't. But the only person who does know everything about your life, your intentions, your amount of ambition is you. Literally no one else in the world can, understand except yourself. That's why the power of self-awareness is so powerful. What's unfortunate is that so many people live the majority of their lives not even know everything about themselves yet. Not, saying I'm perfect myself, but I am open-minded to be aware.

So how do I become more "self-aware?" Well, in the context of this book, there are many ways.

First, know what you want. I hope that if you made it this far into this book, you have a clear understanding of who you are, what you want to be and where you want to go. So first part, check.

Second, know who you surround yourself with. This might take some time for most people, others maybe not so long. This is something not a lot of people tend to be aware about, only because they seem like it's not really something that needs much attention. I mean, friends are friends right? Right. But if you decide to start shifting the dynamic in your daily life to cater to your goals, theoretically speaking, other things that are included in your life will need to be shifted as well. And for you, most likely, that will include your inner circle.

Third, have a clear understanding of how ambitious you are. This part could fall into the grey area a little bit. The awareness of your level of ambition isn't necessarily something they teach you in school or something people use as a conversation starter on a daily basis. However, if you are reading this book and taking it seriously because you actually want to make a difference in your life, it will have to be something that is in the front of your mind all the time, 24/7. You have to constantly ask yourself, "How bad do I actually want this?", "Am I actually doing what I need to do to get where I need to go?" Or my favorite one, "Am I being a little bitch?" Harsh maybe, but practical. Asking these questions to yourself will constantly not only keep you in check, but also keep your ambition level well aware within yourself throughout your daily journey.

What does this have to do with your inner circle? The more aware you are of yourself, the more black and white it will become for you to see who's running with you and who's running in another or opposite direction.

Utilizing the New Era

Even after everything I've said about re-auditing your circle and becoming self-aware to help yourself, that still leaves out a huge aspect in our lives: social media.

Now before we start thinking about social media with a negative connotation, I want to share an interesting perspective.

I am a very optimistic dude and I trained myself to dislike negative outlooks and choose optimism. Why? Because it's practical and it opened my mind to things I wasn't able to before with a negative outlook on everything. Here's what I mean.

Most people in the world look at social media as this thing that changes people and makes people depressed, insecure and overall worse. But in reality, by having an optimistic mindset, I was able to realize that social media isn't a monster, it's a mirror.

What I mean is that your social media channels and profiles are a direct representation of who you are and what your desires are. Why? Because you have total control over every aspect of it. You can follow whoever you want and you can unfollow whoever and whatever you want. If that one influencer makes you feel uncomfortable, unfollow him or her. It's serving as a distraction for you? Oh yeah, so is eating and going out with friends.

So what am I trying to say? I'm saying that if you now understand that social media is a mirror and you have total control over it, you have the choice to choose who you want to surround yourself with even in the digital world. That means re-auditing your followers and following. If there are people you feel that post things that hold you back or get you in a mood or state of mind you don't find beneficial, make the adjustments.

This is a very difficult task to do because not a lot of people have the guts to do it. They like following things that hold them back. They are too lazy to go and make the adjustments.

But let me tell you this, if you were to really adjust who you surround yourself in your social media world, you can really surround yourself with the most inspiring role models in the world every single day. People just one generation ago weren't able to do that, but you can now. Find those people, find those inspirations of yours and keep them close, even if they are on your phone.

The Rhythm Will Save You

Now that you have a clear idea of exactly what actions you need to take in order to be on your way through your journey, the action part of that sentence will be the most difficult part. Action is the bridge between knowledge and success and if you don't take action, guess what you won't have a lot of. So that's where rhythm comes in.

Have you ever memorized something so well only because it had a nice jingle to it? Yes, all the time, right? This will be the same concept we will apply with what I'm about to share with you right now.

When you first start to try to re-audit your circle, it will be the hardest part. The beginning will always be the hardest part. But it's like a snowball, the hardest part is creating it. But once you roll it down the hill, it multiplies by size with minimal effort.

So if that's the case, the more you start to cut people off, unfollow people on Instagram and really take action, it should get easier right? Correct. But I don't want to leave you there.

Here's a system that has helped me in my journey starting off that I believe can be valuable to you too.

When you first commit yourself to finding this rhythm of re-auditing your circle and progressing forward with the right people and influences in your life, the first thing I want you to do is go on all your social media channels and go to your following for each. You would think I would put people first, but let's be honest, the first thing you're going to do on your free time is check your Instagram or Facebook and then make plans with friends or family.

So whether they're Facebook friends, Instagram following, YouTube subscriptions, etc. Go to where you can see the entire list of all of them and scroll through the whole lists and literally ask yourself this person is benefitting you to your goal. And be honest with yourself. If you have an aunt that you like her posts and it inspires you to keep going based off of her cooking posts then knock yourself out and keep her. But what I'm more concerned about are the people you follow that distract, influence you in the opposite direction of your ambition and ultimately hold you back in anyway possible.

This may seem like an extreme tactic for some, but if you're looking for practical and impactful value that can change the course of your life for the better, this is what you do. Plus, let's face it, our social lives are only increasing whether we like it or not. It's how the world develops. So might as well accept that and get ahead of 90% of everyone else and really have control.

So after you got your social life on lock down, have total control and you feel comfortable with no friction in your feed of holding you back, next, let's get to the people that actually pop up in your real life.

This will be a lot harder because it brings everything to the next level of uncomfortability for most. But that's ok, we like adversity, right?

So taking into consideration of how different everyone's social life is, I want to expand this part of the system a little more so it can better serve you. Take one full week and try to take mental, or even physical, note on who appears in your life the most and who are the closest. Now, to be straight up, apply the same concept with your social media re-auditing with these people after the full week is over.

Again, everyone's life is very different and I understand that. So if you do this and it turns out that no one is holding you back and all you feel and see is support from everyone in your circle, then props to you, you are ahead of most. But for most of us, there will be that one person or couple people that you know are holding you back but you just thought it was too extreme to do what you feel you need to do in order to reach your goal.

Don't get it twisted, I'm not saying go up to these people and say something like, "Hey, I got a lot of stuff to work on for myself so I might not be popping up around as much as I usually do." Life is life. If they give you shit for it, then that only reassures your decision on them.

It will not be easy. Especially if it's someone close to you like a family member or long-term friend. When I did this, I literally went through all of my group chats and said the exact same thing. You will have those who still support but some will have those who get caught off guard. Nonetheless, you gotta do what you gotta do. Match your ambitions with your actions- wherever you know your level is.

CHAPTER 5

FUCK 1ST QUARTER HIGHS

Alright, we got all the tools, we're rubbing our hands together ready to go. Maybe some of us have already started. But after all these tactics, valuable information and maybe even motivation, there is one more thing that we cannot leave out no matter what. The insane thing is that this one last concept is the one concept that 98% of people that start this journey for themselves lack. I'm talking about the long term.

Now before you start exploding in your head about how fucking cliche that sounds, it is the utmost important aspect within this whole entire book. Why? Because understanding what I'm about to share with you has the power to impact the rest of your life or just the next two months, like all the other times you may have attempted this journey.

This perspective will be the core foundation of whether you reach your breakthrough or not and I am more than willing to share it with you only if you are just as willing. If you are not as willing, it will not make an impact in your life in any way whatsoever. So if you're ready, let's finish strong.

1st Quarter Highs

In NBA basketball, there are four quarters. Each quarter being 12 minutes long. First I want to talk about the players that tend to be on a roll for the first quarter. They blast it 100% and get all the rebounds, all the three pointers, they basically look like the all-star of the game. And then second quarter comes. Then the third. Now the fourth. Sadly, the player that I'm using as an example isn't Kobe, Lebron, Jordan, or any other all-star. He's a rookie. So if that's the case, what do you think he looks like now in the fourth quarter?

For this hypothetical situation, not so well. As most rookies would be. What am I trying to say? I'm saying that most of the people in this world and even in our own lives do things in the short term rather than the long term. They'd rather receive the high for the first quarter than to win the game and get the ultimate applause.

I don't blame them though. It's typical human nature to lean towards instant gratitude. But the question you have to ask yourself is do you really want to be like every other typical human? This isn't a trick question. If you actually do, than keep doing you. But now that you're aware of your level of ambition, how much are you going to start focusing on the long term rather than the short term?

What does this short term vs long term thing have to do with my fitness journey in the first place? Because short term behavior leads to short term results. And we're not here to get short term results. So what is this short term behavior you have to avoid in order to last? Let's find out.

Don't Let Opinions Deceive You

Let me provide more context. Caring about opinions is a huge vulnerability and pure short term behavior. Here's why.

Opinions aren't necessarily a bad, but they could be. Opinions have the power to steer you off course no matter if they're good opinions or bad opinions. Good ones too?! Yes. Let me give you some examples. You create a painting took you months. You put your blood sweat and tears into it. Your hands are all blistered from the brushes. You gave it your all. You show it to your friend for the first time. She says, "Oh this is really awesome, you're honestly the best!" But later in the day, you find out through a mutual friend that she actually thought it was just alright. Fuck. That messes with your head. Why should you make another one. You know it's your passion but why should you continue if it's just going to be "alright" to people?

Let's say she meant it, both times. You got that recognition. You got that high. You now believe that you're the shit.

But now you're all up in your feels, you feel like you should treat yourself and take a longer break. That longer break turns into two breaks because you feel like you already know you can beast it. And now you're not painting as much as you usually do. You're comfortable. You don't feel the need to improve yourself because everyone now is telling you that you're "the shit". Congrats, you're passion just plateaued. So what do we do with opinions?

Three words. Close your ears. When you go along your journey, especially after a while, you will receive a lot of opinions. Some being positive, some being negative. But at the end of the day, fuck everyones opinion. Stay on your course. Don't crushed by them, but don't get high on your own supply by them either. Know where you are in your game and keep grinding. That's the key.

So many people do it for the attention and opinions of others but now they allowed the opinions to have control over their actions, therefore, limiting their goals. Don't get tempted. Stay humble and stay confident. Someone says you fucking suck and you don't know what you're doing? Take a step back, reassess where you actually are because you're the only one who knows the 100% context of your own life and you know the truth, and move past it.

People leaving comments on your posts that you're killing it and you're a beast? Appreciate it. But understand where you are in your own game and realize that you still have a lot to learn and a long ways to go.

I couldn't emphasize how crucial this mindset is. Too

many people do it for the opinions and give up because of other people's actual fucking opinion. Fuck opinions, play your game. If you manage to pull this off, you will last and will never fall short of the 2 month cliff ever again.

Micro For Macro

We're talking a lot of long term game and I understand that that's not a very easy thing to hear. We want results tomorrow, we don't want to be patient, we want the instant gratitude. Even though that's just how it is, I want to try to fill in some of the cracks and provide more context to ultimately get your head 100% clear of what mindset you need to have in order to make this ideal lifestyle of yours a true reality and not some scheme just to get you to pay for a book.

Micro for macro is the most basic, black and white summary of how I want you to think on a daily basis. So what does it mean?

You want to accomplish the micro tasks in order to produce the macro result. You want to prepare all the ingredients properly in order to cook the meal. These include all the small, tedious tasks that the average person would skip over and not put much attention to such as skipping eating out, cutting off that one acquaintance that constantly keeps tempting you to delay your ambition and even not pressing the snooze button when you know you only have time to workout in the morning because of work or school.

I hate to put it this way but they really do add up. And if you half-ass your ingredients, you're going to get a half-ass meal and I'm not here to prepare you for a half-ass meal. I want help you prepare to produce real results and actually leave an impact in your life.

So everyday, I want you to see these small things, these small adjustments and actions as a single puzzle piece to your ultimate creation and for every piece that you choose to skip, the uglier the end product will look like.

This is your chance. This is your opportunity to actually make a change for yourself. You know what to eat and how to eat it. You know to increase the intensity to your ambition level and to not give yourself excuses to not raise the bar higher when you need to. You have all the tools around your hip. What are you going to do with them?

Most people that read this book will get hyped up for the first week and then forget everything and go back to the old ways. No doubt about it. But will you be one of those people?

You know to think for the long term now and that the 1st quarter highs no longer hold value for you. You don't care about others' opinions, you won't alter your path just because someone insults you. You won't. It's not worth it anymore.

You want to change. You want to be optimistic for your future, and for some, for the future of your family and kids. This is your time. No one else is going to make you do anything. Only you and you.

I promise you, if you manage to pull this off, which I believe that you can and you will, you will be able to live the rest of your life truly happy. So much so that if you were to die the next day, you will be satisfied with what you accomplished. No matter how many times you had to reject fried food. No matter how many temptations and struggles you face. It would finally all be worth it to you at the end.

I want that for you. I'm not creating this book for your money. I'm creating this book with the hopes that the value and information in this book could be available to you and you can take it and really change the course of your life with it. That's it. Nothing else.

If there is no one else in your life that believes you can do it and you feel that you have no support, I want you to know that I believe 100% that you can kill it and make that change. No matter how much time passes on after you close this book. I believe you can. Any human can.

Don't get sucked into the short term, I want to see you succeed in the long term. You got it.

www.ingramcontent.com/pod-product-compliance
Lightning Source LLC
Chambersburg PA
CBHW051123250726
48655CB00007B/2856